TUI NAI MESSAGE

FOR NOVICES

Discover Ancient Wisdom For Healing, Balance, Personal Transformation, Overcoming Adversity, And Building A Resilient Future Through The Power Of Tui Nai

DR. TADEO KASEN

Table of Contents

DISCLIAMER

This book is intended for informational and educational purposes only. The content provided in this book is not a substitute for professional medical advice, diagnosis, or treatment. Always seek the advice of your physician or other qualified health provider with any questions you may have regarding a medical condition.

The techniques and practices described in this book are based on general principles and may not be suitable for everyone. Individual results may vary, and it is important to consult with a qualified healthcare professional before undertaking any new health or wellness program.

The author and publisher of this book are not responsible for any adverse effects or consequences resulting from the use of information, suggestions, exercises, or techniques presented herein. The reader assumes full responsibility for his or her actions and choices. The information provided in this book is accurate and reliable. However, the author and publisher make no representation or warranties of any kind, express or implied, regarding the completeness, accuracy, reliability, or suitability of the information provided.

Any References to specific products, services, or organizations do not imply endorsement or recommendation by the author.

By reading this book, the reader acknowledges and agrees to the terms of this disclaimer. If the reader does not agree with these terms, they should not use the information provided in this book.

CHAPTER ONE

Tui Na Massage Fundamentals

Tui Na, a traditional Chinese massage technique, has a long history extending back thousands of years. Tui Na, which is based on traditional Chinese medicine, strives to restore the balance of energy inside the body to improve general health and well-being. This therapeutic massage combines rhythmic compression, acupressure, and stretching methods to create a one-of-a-kind and powerful healing therapy.

Tui Na's Origins

Tui Na may be traced back to ancient China, where it originated as an essential component of traditional Chinese medicine (TCM). Tui Na's foundations are strongly rooted in the yin and yang principles, as well as the idea of Qi (pronounced "chee"), the vital energy that runs through the body's meridians.

Tui Na's history is intertwined with that of traditional Chinese medicine, which encompasses acupuncture, herbal medicine, and other therapeutic methods. Tui Na was first documented during the Shang Dynasty (approximately 1700-1027 BCE) when it was described in ancient books as a means of treatment. Tui Na has evolved throughout the years, combining ideas from Taoist philosophy and other ancient Chinese therapeutic methods.

Tui Na was refined and systematized further throughout the Ming (1368-1644) and Qing (1644-1912) periods. Skilled practitioners began to codify Tui Na techniques and ideas, helping it to evolve as a unique and acknowledged therapeutic practice within the larger landscape of traditional Chinese medicine.

Tui Na, despite its profound historical roots, encountered obstacles during China's numerous eras of modernization. However, Tui Na's persistent efficacy, along with the expanding global interest in alternative and complementary medicines, has led to a resurgence of interest in modern times. Tui Na is now used not only in China but increasingly across the world, as people seek holistic methods to health and wellness.

Tui Na Principles And Concepts

Tui Na is founded on several core ideas and concepts derived from traditional Chinese medicine. The belief that the body's health is impacted by the balance and flow of Qi, the essential life force, is central to its philosophy. Disruptions in the flow of Qi, according to TCM, cause imbalances and, ultimately, sickness. Tui Na seeks to restore this equilibrium by manipulating the energy pathways and acupoints of the body.

Tui Na incorporates the notion of Yin and Yang, which symbolize conflicting yet complementary energies in the cosmos. Practitioners strive to create balance by balancing the Yin and Yang components of the body. Tui Na acknowledges that imbalances in these energies can appear as physical or emotional disorders, and the massage methods are intended to correct these imbalances.

Tui Na emphasizes the relevance of the meridian system in addition to Qi, Yin, and Yang. Meridians are energy routes that link numerous organs and tissues throughout the body. Tui Na practitioners use their understanding of these meridians to target specific sites and channels, aiding healing and enabling the smooth flow of energy.

Tui Na Techniques

Tui Na uses a variety of techniques that set it apart from other types of massage treatment. These techniques are intended to manipulate Qi and encourage free energy flow throughout the body. "Anmo," a sort of pressing and rubbing that increases the flow of Qi in the meridians, is one of the fundamental methods.

Another important component of Tui Na is the use of the terms "Tui" and "Na," which relate to pushing and gripping methods, respectively. Tui is characterized by rhythmic pushing movements, whereas Na is characterized by gripping and raising. These techniques are used to reduce tension, promote circulation, and restore balance at certain acupoints and meridians.

Acupressure is a key component of Tui Na, with practitioners applying pressure to particular acupoints in the body's meridians with their fingers, palms, or elbows. This pressure increases the flow of Qi and can help relieve pain and promote relaxation.

Tui Na also includes stretching and joint manipulation. These approaches attempt to improve flexibility, relieve muscle and joint tension, and increase the total range of motion. Tui Na massage targets particular concerns while also promoting a sense of overall well-being by including flexibility in the massage.

To summarize, Tui Na massage is a time-honored therapeutic method rooted in ancient Chinese medicine. Its ideas and concepts, which are based on a knowledge of Qi, Yin, and Yang, as well as the meridian system, serve as the cornerstone of its holistic approach to health and wellbeing.

Tui Na practices, such as Anmo, Tui, Na, acupressure, and stretching, work together to restore balance, relieve pain, and encourage the free flow of energy throughout the body. As Tui Na grows in popularity across the world, its ancient knowledge and efficient healing practices add to the diversified landscape of holistic healthcare.

Tui Na Massage Advantages

Tui Na, a type of traditional Chinese massage, has grown in popularity across the world due to its therapeutic effects. Tui Na is a Traditional Chinese Medicine (TCM) technique that focuses on harmonizing the flow of Qi (vital energy) in the body. Various hand movements, including pressing, tugging, kneading, and stretching, are used to boost the body's natural healing processes. Here are some of the most important advantages of Tui Na massage:

1. Tui Na is well-known for its ability to alleviate both acute and chronic pain. Practitioners can relieve muscle tension, decrease inflammation, and improve

blood circulation by targeting certain acupoints and meridians. Tui Na is therefore an ideal alternative for anyone suffering from illnesses such as arthritis, back pain, and migraines.

2. Stress Reduction: Tui Na relieves not only physical suffering but also mental and emotional stress. The massage's rhythmic and relaxing methods encourage relaxation and aid in the release of muscular tension. Tui Na is a comprehensive therapy for relieving stress-related illnesses due to this dual approach.

3. Improved Circulation: The manipulative techniques used in Tui Na increase blood circulation, allowing oxygen and nutrients to move more freely throughout the body. This improved circulation not only improves general health but also hastens the body's natural healing processes.

4. Tui Na incorporates stretches and joint mobilizations, which contribute to increased flexibility and range of motion. This is especially

advantageous for people who have musculoskeletal disorders since it helps restore and maintain healthy joint function.

5. Tui Na is said to improve the immune system by regulating the body's energy and increasing the flow of Qi. Regular sessions may help to greater resilience to diseases and faster recovery from a variety of health difficulties.

6. Digestive Health: In TCM, digestive disorders are frequently connected to energy imbalances in the body. Tui Na massage can help to correct these imbalances by concentrating on digestive acupoints. This can help relieve indigestion, bloating, and constipation problems.

7. Tui Na stimulates the lymphatic system, which aids in the evacuation of toxins from the body. This massage method aids the body's natural detoxification processes by encouraging waste product removal.

8. Tui Na works to balance the flow of energy via the body's meridians, ensuring that Qi is distributed appropriately. This equilibrium is critical for general health and avoiding the advent of many diseases.

9. Enhanced Sleep Quality: Many people report increased sleep quality following Tui Na sessions. Massage relaxation, along with its stress-relieving benefits, can significantly alter sleep patterns and lead to a more peaceful night.

10. Tui Na is a holistic therapy that targets the mind and soul as well as the body. This massage style coincides with the holistic principles of Traditional Chinese Medicine by fostering bodily harmony, leading to overall well-being.

CHAPTER TWO

Contraindications And Indications

While Tui Na has many health advantages, it is important to examine both indications (when it is suggested) and contraindications (when it should be avoided) to guarantee the massage's safety and efficacy.

Indications:

1. Tui Na is especially beneficial for disorders involving musculoskeletal discomfort, such as arthritis, back pain, and muscular strains.

2. Individuals suffering from stress, anxiety, or tension might benefit from Tui Na's soothing and stress-relieving benefits.

3. Tui Na's mix of massage and joint mobilization makes it appropriate for resolving joint issues and enhancing range of motion.

4. Digestive Disorders: Tui Na is recommended for people who have digestive problems since it can assist in regulating energy flow in the digestive tract.

5. Headaches and Migraines: Tui Na's therapeutic techniques make it a feasible alternative for relieving headaches and migraines, which are frequently related to tension and stress.

6. Insomnia: Tui Na's capacity to promote relaxation and balance energy might help individuals who suffer from insomnia sleep better.

7. Immune System Support: People who want to improve their immune system function may find Tui Na useful for general health.

Contraindications:

1. While moderate massage is typically regarded safe during pregnancy, more powerful Tui Na methods may be contraindicated, particularly in the first trimester.

2. Tui Na should be avoided in regions where there are active infections or skin disorders to prevent the spread of the infection.

3. Fractures or Severe Injuries: Tui Na may not be useful in situations of severe injuries or fractures until the initial acute phase has passed.

4. Direct manipulation over open wounds or burns is not recommended to prevent the worsening of the damage and potential infection.

5. Individuals with significant medical issues, such as cardiovascular disease or cancer, should see their healthcare professional before undertaking Tui Na or any type of massage treatment.

6. If a person has a contagious sickness, it is best to postpone Tui Na to avoid spreading the infection to the practitioner or other customers.

Tui Na Vs. Other Massage Methods

Tui Na is distinguished from other massage treatments by its concepts, techniques, and holistic approach. Here's a comparison between Tui Na and other common massage techniques:

1. Tui Na vs. Swedish Massage: Which Is Better?

• Techniques: Tui Na massage combines kneading, rolling, and stretching, whereas Swedish massage focuses on long, flowing strokes and circular motions.

• Goal: Tui Na focuses on Qi balance and specific health issues, whereas Swedish massage tries to relax muscles and enhance circulation.

2. Tui Na vs. Deep Tissue Massage: Which Is Better?

• Pressure: Tui Na employs a range of pressures, including lighter approaches for energy balance and deeper pressure for addressing specific difficulties.

Deep tissue massage employs sustained, strong pressure to relieve chronic muscular tension.

• Approach: Tui Na incorporates joint mobilizations and stretches, whereas deep tissue massage focuses on muscle layers.

3. Shiatsu vs. Tui Na:

• methods: Tui Na uses a larger range of methods, including as rolling and stretching, whereas Shiatsu largely involves finger pressure on particular acupoints.

• Tui Na is based on TCM principles and addresses both physical and energetic abnormalities. While Shiatsu originated in Japan, it shares the principles of meridians and acupoints.

4. Tui Na vs. Thai Massage: Which Is Better?

• Clothes: Tui Na is normally conducted on a clothed or draped client, whereas Thai massage is performed on a mat with the client wearing loose garments.

Stretching is used in both modalities, although Thai massage is noted for its extensive use of passive stretching.

5. Tui Na vs. Reflexology: Which Is Better?

• Concentration: Tui Na treats the entire body, including the muscles and joints, whereas reflexology concentrates on particular reflex sites on the feet, hands, and ears.

• Methodology: Tui Na includes direct manipulation of soft tissues, whereas reflexology involves applying pressure to particular locations said to correlate to organs and systems.

Traditional Chinese Medicine And Tui Na

Tui Na is profoundly ingrained in the framework of Traditional Chinese Medicine (TCM), sharing its fundamental principles and promoting comprehensive recovery. Here's how Tui Na relates to major TCM concepts:

1. Meridians and Qi:

• Traditional Chinese Medicine (TCM) Perspective: Tui Na is based on the idea that health is maintained when Qi flows easily through the body's meridians. Qi imbalances can cause a variety of health problems.

• Tui Na Application: Tui Na practitioners employ particular techniques to manipulate Qi, encouraging balance and removing meridians obstructions.

2. Yang and Yin:

TCM emphasizes the balance of Yin and Yang, which reflect opposing yet complementary forces. When these factors are in balance, health results.

• Tui Na Application: Tui Na tries to restore balance by recognizing and correcting Yin and Yang imbalances in the body.

3. Five Components:

• TCM Perspective: The Five Elements theory divides the body's organs and tissues into Wood, Fire, Earth, Metal, and Water, each with its own set of characteristics.

• Tui Na Treatments: Tui Na treatments are targeted to correct imbalances connected to certain elements, fostering harmony and restoring balance.

4. Diagnosis based on Pulse and Tongue:

• TCM Perspective: TCM practitioners examine the status of Qi, Blood, and Yin-Yang within the body using pulse and tongue diagnostic.

• Tui Na Application: Tui Na practitioners may use pulse and tongue analysis to personalize the massage to the individual's particular health needs.

5. Holistic Wellness and Prevention:

• TCM Perspective: TCM emphasizes preventative medicine and holistic well-being, treating the underlying causes of imbalance before symptoms appear.

• Tui Na Application: Tui Na complements this preventative strategy by encouraging general well-being and resolving imbalances early on.

Finally, Tui Na massage provides a unique combination of therapeutic effects based on Traditional Chinese Medicine concepts. Its holistic approach, which combines physical manipulation with an emphasis on energy flow, distinguishes it from other massage treatments. Understanding the indications and contraindications ensures that people may experience the many benefits of Tui Na safely while comparing it to other massage modalities emphasizes its uniqueness. Tui Na's incorporation within the larger framework of Traditional Chinese Medicine emphasizes its importance in fostering balance, harmony, and overall well-being.

CHAPTER THREE

Tui Na Massage Training And Certification

Tui Na massage, a traditional Chinese bodywork therapy, is becoming increasingly popular due to its therapeutic effects. Adequate training and certification are required to become a skilled Tui Na practitioner. Tui Na training programs include both theoretical and practical abilities, ensuring that practitioners have a thorough understanding of this ancient healing practice.

Tui Na training often includes a study of Traditional Chinese Medicine (TCM) principles, as Tui Na is closely related to TCM ideas such as Qi (vital energy), meridians, and Yin-Yang balance. Prospective practitioners learn about the energy flow of the body as well as the significance of acupressure sites in supporting general well-being. Understanding these fundamental concepts is essential for successful Tui Na practice.

Tui Na certification frequently entails completing a planned program that may include TCM theory, anatomy, and hands-on Tui Na practices. Many training programs additionally demand that students complete a specified number of supervised practice hours. This hands-on experience is crucial for polishing abilities and developing the sensitivity required to deal with the energy and bodily structure of a client.

Certification in traditional Chinese medicine or Tui Na can be obtained from approved organizations. Certification certifies a practitioner's abilities while also assuring clients of their competence and adherence to professional norms. Practitioners must select renowned training programs and certification authorities to guarantee they obtain excellent education and industry recognition.

Tui Na practice also emphasizes ongoing education. Continuous learning, like in any expanding profession, keeps practitioners up to speed on new techniques, research, and breakthroughs in Tui Na and related fields. Workshops, seminars, and advanced training courses allow practitioners to expand their knowledge and enhance their abilities, which contributes to their professional development.

Tui Na Integration Into Wellness Practices

Tui Na massage, with its emphasis on balancing the body's energy and supporting natural healing, fits in flawlessly with wellness practices. Tui Na, when included in wellness practices, provides a comprehensive approach to health, treating both physical and energetic elements. Tui Na can improve wellness habits in the following ways:

1. Tui Na is well-known for its ability to alleviate tension and induce relaxation. Individuals can find respite from the physical and emotional strains of daily living by adopting Tui Na into their health habits. Tui Na's gentle yet strong manipulations assist in relieving muscular tension and promote Qi flow, encouraging a sense of serenity and well-being.

2. Tui Na is beneficial in treating a variety of pain issues, including musculoskeletal pain, headaches, and chronic illnesses. Integrating Tui Na into health routines can be especially useful for anyone looking for natural, non-invasive pain relief. Tui Na's tailored methods treat particular areas of discomfort, bringing pain alleviation and better mobility.

3. Tui Na focuses on regulating the body's energy, and adding it into health routines helps to regulate Qi flow. This energy balance is necessary for good health and vigor. Individuals may assist their body's natural ability to heal and maintain homeostasis by including Tui Na in their wellness routines, adding to long-term well-being.

4. Improved Circulation: Tui Na massage improves blood circulation and lymphatic drainage. This can help with improved nutrition and oxygen supply to cells, as well as more effective waste elimination from the body. Tui Na incorporates wellness practices to improve overall circulatory health and supports the body's important processes.

5. Tui Na can be used in conjunction with other health techniques such as yoga, meditation, and nutritional treatment. Combining Tui Na with other holistic therapies creates a holistic approach to well-being that addresses the physical, mental, and energetic components of health.

Examples Of Tui Na Massage

Case studies give useful insights into the practical application and efficacy of Tui Na massage in resolving a variety of health concerns. These real-world examples demonstrate Tui Na's adaptability and potential influence on people's well-being. Here are a few case studies demonstrating Tui Na's usefulness in various scenarios:

1. Chronic Pain Management: A middle-aged man with chronic lower back pain sought Tui Na therapy after failing to find relief from other conventional therapies. The Tui Na practitioner used acupressure, kneading, and stretching techniques to target the problem region. The client reported considerable pain reduction and better mobility throughout a

series of sessions, demonstrating Tui Na's effectiveness in addressing chronic musculoskeletal disorders.

2. Tension and Anxiety Reduction: To combat high levels of tension and anxiety, a young professional added frequent Tui Na sessions into their health routine. Tui Na's relaxing effects, along with its capacity to release tension, resulted in a considerable drop in stress levels. The customer experienced better sleep, a better mood, and a stronger overall sensation of calm.

3. Headache Relief: A client with chronic tension headaches sought Tui Na therapy to address the underlying muscular tension that was causing their headaches. The Tui Na practitioner concentrated on acupressure sites associated with headache alleviation and used methods to relax the neck and shoulders. After a few sessions, the client reported a considerable reduction in the frequency and intensity of headaches.

4. Tui Na's impact on the digestive system was obvious in an instance when a client with digestive disorders focused on abdominal Tui Na massage. Techniques were used by the practitioner to accelerate digestion and improve the smooth passage of Qi in the abdominal region. The customer noticed better digestion, less bloating, and overall digestive well-being.

5. Post-Injury Rehabilitation: Tui Na assisted in the rehabilitation of a person recuperating from a sports injury. The treatments were targeted to address particular regions impacted by the injury, with Tui Na methods used to improve blood circulation, decrease inflammation, and promote tissue recovery. Tui Na helped the client recover faster and with a greater range of motion, demonstrating Tui Na's ability to aid in rehabilitation efforts.

To summarize, Tui Na massage is a wonderful complement to health practices due to its rich history and therapeutic effects. Practitioners who get sufficient training and certification can learn the art of Tui Na and contribute to the well-being of those seeking natural and holistic approaches to health. Tui Na's incorporation into wellness routines, along with case study research, demonstrates its usefulness in resolving a wide range of health conditions and increasing overall balance and vitality.

CHAPTER FOUR

Tui Na Massage Research And Study

Tui Na, a traditional Chinese therapeutic massage, is gaining popularity in both the East and the West because of its potential health advantages. Through scientific investigations, academics and practitioners have dug into understanding the mechanics and benefits of Tui Na massage over the years. This study looked at a variety of facets of Tui Na, from its physiological influence on the body to its usefulness in treating certain illnesses.

One field of study focuses on the physiological changes brought about by Tui Na massage. Tui Na has been shown in studies to influence the autonomic nervous system, resulting in a decrease in stress hormones such as cortisol and an increase in parasympathetic activity.

This shows that Tui Na has a soothing and stress-relieving impact on the body, which contributes to its potential as a holistic approach to healing.

Furthermore, studies have looked at the effects of Tui Na on various health issues. For example, studies have looked into its effectiveness in treating musculoskeletal disorders like chronic neck pain and lower back pain.

The results have been promising, with Tui Na producing comparable or even better results than traditional treatments such as medication or physical therapy. This suggests that Tui Na could be an effective alternative or complementary therapy for people suffering from musculoskeletal problems.

Tui Na has also been studied for its effects on the circulatory and immune systems. According to research, the massage technique may improve blood circulation and immune function.

These findings suggest that Tui Na may play a role in promoting overall health and preventing illnesses.

Tui Na has been studied for its psychological benefits in addition to its physiological effects. Tui Na massage has been shown in studies to improve mental health by lowering anxiety and depression levels. During a massage session, the combination of physical manipulation and focused attention may contribute to a sense of relaxation and emotional balance.

However, while there is a growing body of research supporting the benefits of Tui Na, more high-quality studies is needed to definitively establish its effectiveness for specific conditions. Researchers continue to struggle with standardizing Tui Na protocols, variations in practitioner skills, and the need for larger sample sizes as they seek a more comprehensive understanding of Tui Na's therapeutic potential.

Tui Na Massage's Cultural Importance

Tui Na massage has its origins in Chinese culture and traditional Chinese medicine (TCM). Its roots can be traced back thousands of years, and its practice is intertwined with the philosophical principles that serve as TCM's foundation.

Understanding the cultural significance of Tui Na necessitates investigating its historical context, philosophical underpinnings, and role in promoting body balance and harmony.

The body is viewed as an interconnected system of energy, or "qi," flowing through meridians in traditional Chinese medicine. Tui Na is intended to control the flow of qi, thereby promoting balance and harmony. It follows the same principles as acupuncture and herbal medicine and is an essential component of TCM's holistic approach to health and well-being.

Tui Na's cultural significance extends beyond its theoretical framework. It is deeply ingrained in Chinese daily life and medical practices. Tui Na is not only a therapeutic modality in China, but it is also accepted as a form of preventive medicine. Many people incorporate Tui Na into their daily routine to maintain health and prevent imbalances from manifesting as illnesses. This cultural perspective emphasizes the idea that Tui Na is more than just a treatment for ailments; it is also a way to promote overall wellness.

Furthermore, Tui Na has cultural significance in terms of family and community. Tui Na techniques are frequently passed down through generations in traditional Chinese households, creating a familial connection to this healing practice. Tui Na techniques may be practiced differently by different families, preserving a cultural heritage that goes beyond textbooks and formal training.

The cultural significance of Tui Na can also be seen in its role in Chinese festivals and celebrations. Tui Na practitioners may offer their services to promote health and well-being in the community during traditional festivals and important events. Tui Na's communal aspect emphasizes its role as a shared cultural experience as well as an individual therapeutic practice.

Tui Na's cultural significance has begun to transcend its Chinese origins as it grows in popularity around the world. Many people from various cultural backgrounds are now embracing Tui Na as an important part of their wellness routine, praising its holistic approach and alignment with principles of balance and harmony.

Tui Na Massage Future Trends

Tui Na Massage's future is being defined by a blend of traditional knowledge, scientific investigation, and global integration. As interest in holistic and alternative therapies grows, various tendencies emerge that represent the changing environment of Tui Na and its role in modern healthcare.

The incorporation of Tui Na into conventional healthcare procedures is one prominent trend. Tui Na is rapidly being acknowledged as a legitimate supplementary therapy for a variety of health issues as research continues to substantiate its therapeutic advantages. Healthcare practitioners are looking into incorporating Tui Na into treatment programs to develop a more integrative approach that mixes mainstream medicine with traditional healing practices.

Technological improvements are also having an impact on the future of Tui Na. Tui Na practitioners may now reach a worldwide audience through virtual platforms and telemedicine services. Individuals may enjoy the advantages of this traditional massage from the comfort of their own homes thanks to online Tui Na sessions led by professional practitioners. This development is consistent with the overall shift toward digital health and wellness offerings.

Furthermore, Tui Na is making a comeback in spa and wellness environments. Spas are introducing Tui Na into their service offerings as people seek holistic ways of relaxation and renewal.

Tui Na combined with other wellness activities like yoga and meditation shows a rising understanding of the interdependence of physical, mental, and spiritual well-being.

Tui Na's future is likewise being shaped by education and professionalization. As the need for skilled practitioners grows, regulated training programs and certification are becoming more important. This step toward professionalization not only assures a greater level of competence among practitioners, but also helps to integrate Tui Na into official healthcare settings.

Furthermore, Tui Na research is anticipated to increase, filling present gaps in understanding and giving a stronger evidence-based foundation. High-quality research on Tui Na's unique mechanisms, ideal uses, and long-term benefits will help to a better understanding of this ancient therapy.

Finally, the future of Tui Na massage looks promising as it bridges the gap between ancient knowledge and modern treatment. Tui Na's incorporation into mainstream practices, technology improvements, rebirth in wellness settings, and emphasis on teaching and research all contribute to Tui Na's developing environment in the years ahead.

41

Conclusion

Finally, the Tui Na massage, which is based on traditional Chinese medicine, provides a comprehensive approach to well-being by balancing the body's essential energy, or Qi. Tui Na attempts to restore balance and promote natural healing via the expert manipulation of pressure points, stretching, and rhythmic motions. This therapeutic massage goes beyond simple relaxation by addressing particular health conditions and attempting to correct both physical and energy imbalances.

Tui Na's success stems from its capacity to improve blood circulation, relieve stress, and boost the body's self-healing capabilities. Individuals who experience the relaxing benefits of Tui Na frequently find alleviation from a variety of diseases, including muscular pain, tension, and exhaustion. Furthermore, Tui Na promotes a profound mind-body connection, resulting in a sensation of calm and refreshment.

Tui Na massage has promise for people seeking a natural and holistic approach to wellbeing, whether utilized as a single therapy or in conjunction with other types of healthcare.

Tui Na is a great modality for maintaining health and balance in our fast-paced world because of its rich history and time-tested techniques, which continue to resonate in current wellness practices. Embracing Tui Na concepts opens the door to long-lasting health and a revitalized sense of vibrancy.